10240631

ROBERT COCKS & CO.'S MODERN METHODS.—No. 12.

Learn to Breathe and Control your Breath;
Learn also to Increase the Power and Beautify the Quality of your Voice; by Studying

TWELVE LESSONS ON BREATHING AND BREATH CONTROL:

FOR

Singers, Speakers, and Teachers.

BY

GEORGE E. THORP.

Author of "Colour Audition and its Relation to Voice Production," and co-Author of "A Text-Book on the Natural Use of the Voice."

These Lessons are so written that you can, by studying them, master the fundamental principles employed in the use of the voice

WITHOUT A MASTER.

PRICE 1/-

INTRODUCTION.

ALTHOUGH there are many works treating of the act of respiration, there is not one, so far as I know, which is in itself a practical teacher of this most important subject.

The object of these lessons is four-fold. First, to point out in what respects inspiration is, in nearly every case, defective; second, to correct defective breathing; third, to develop the chest and lungs to their fullest extent; and fourth, to show how to control the breath when it is used for the purposes of phonation and articulation.

These lessons are intended not only for singers and speakers, but also for those who teach children, because the largest and healthiest growth of the body, as well as the greatest development of the voice, is attained only through the practice of full and unimpeded respiration.

GEORGE E. THORP.

10, Prince's-street, Hanover-square,
London, W. Jan. 1896.

TWELVE LESSONS
ON
BREATHING
AND
BREATH CONTROL.

LESSON I.

IN BREATHING.

BREATHING is a natural function which, when not perverted or misguided, is the same in man and woman. These lessons, therefore, are applicable to both. Their object is, first, to enable the student to get an accurate knowledge of what he does in *ordinary breathing*; second, to correct bad habits, if they have been acquired, and at the same time to develop his lung capacity.

A STUDY OF THE MOVEMENTS IN ORDINARY INSPIRATION.

MASTER. What movements of the chest and upper part of the abdomen do you feel when taking a full breath?

PUPIL. I find it rather difficult to answer that question, some of the movements being uncertain.

MASTER. Very well, if I ask a few leading questions perhaps you will find it less difficult. Place one of your hands on the abdomen at the waist line, and tell me whether it moves in or out as you fill the lungs.

PUPIL. It moved outward a little.

MASTER. Later on, when you have learned to breathe correctly, I shall ask you about the movement of the abdomen again, and compare your answer with the one just given. Now place your hands on your sides, just above the waist line, and describe the movement of the ribs as you inspire.

PUPIL. The ribs moved outward a very little.

MASTER. Again, place one hand on the back immediately above the waist line so that the finger tips touch the spinal column, and the other on the side, also above the waist line, so that the tips of the fingers are directly below the breast-bone, and note whether there is a movement at one or both places as you inspire.

PUPIL. There is a forward movement of the ribs, but it is less than that which I felt at the sides.

MASTER. Do you not also feel a movement of the ribs at the back?

PUPIL. No. I can feel nothing there.

MASTER. Now place the hands on the sides as close up under the arms as possible, and describe the movement there when inspiring.

PUPIL. There is an outward movement of the ribs.

MASTER. How does the movement there compare with that lower down on the sides?

PUPIL. It is much more marked.

MASTER. We have already seen that there was no movement of the ribs low down at the back. Now place your hand on your back well up under the shoulder blade, and see if there is a movement there.

PUPIL. Yes, at that point the ribs appear to swing backward a little.

MASTER. Lastly, I wish you to observe the movements of the upper part of the chest during inspiration. To assist you in this observation, take a small book or ruler about twelve inches long, place one end of it on the top of the breast bone, letting the other end come up before the face, and be nearly parallel with it. Now inspire and observe the movements of the book or ruler.

PUPIL. As I inhale it both rises and moves out from the face.

MASTER. What actions of the chest does that indicate?

PUPIL. It indicates that the chest both rises and moves outward.

MASTER. Now tell me all the movements you have observed for a full inspiration.

PUPIL. I found:

1st, that the *upper part of the abdomen moved out* a little.

2nd, that the *ribs moved out a little at the sides just above the waist line.*

3rd, that they *moved out much more under the arms.*

4th, that they *moved forward at the end of the breast bone.*

5th, that they *moved backward under the shoulderb lades.*

6th, that the *upper part of the chest moved both up and forward.*

This is a record made by a lady before beginning her studies in singing. Each student should make a similar record before beginning these lessons, but he should not expect to feel the movements the same in every respect as they are given above. Most ladies find that the lower ribs move but very little. Gentlemen observe that the movements of the lower part of the ribs are very strongly marked, while the upper part of the chest remains nearly or quite motionless. I would urge each student, not only to make a record of the movements of the chest at each of the points mentioned, but also to *measure* and record those movements. The benefit derived from these lessons will depend upon the development of the muscles used in inspiration, expiration, and breath control.

LESSON II.

IN BREATHING.

WE wish to reach all cases of incorrect breathing, not only to set into motion those muscles which have become inactive, but also to strengthen those which are weak. Therefore, we will divide the inspiratory act into four parts, each of which you are to practise separately.

THE PARTS OF THE ACT OF INSPIRATION ARE:

1st. The lateral or outward movement of the ribs.
2nd. The backward movement of the ribs.
3rd. The upward movement of the ribs.
4th. The forward movement of the ribs.

Before beginning the practice of these exercises *remove all close-fitting garments.* By *close-fitting* garments I mean *all those garments in which the ribs cannot expand, that is, swing in and out a distance of four inches from fullest inspiration to fullest expiration.*

While practising these exercises (and usually in singing) breath should enter the lungs through the nose. When inhaled in this way the air passes over the vocal chords and into the lungs both *filtered, moistened*, and *warmed*. The small hairs of the nose filter the air, the mucus which covers the mucous membrane moistens it, and the numerous blood-vessels just below the surface of the membrane warm the air as it passes through into the pharynx, and further on into the lungs. These three conditions of the air are necessary to preserve a healthy state of vocal organs and lungs.

THE LATERAL EXPANSION AND ITS DEVELOPMENT.

MASTER. Place one hand on your chest below the chin, the other on the side just above the waist line, and, *without allowing the chest to rise*, take a short, deep breath. How does this lateral expansion of the ribs compare with their expansion when breathing as you usually do?

PUPIL. I find the movement much greater when taking the short, deep breath, but is such breathing natural?

MASTER. Let us see. Observe your friend speaking excitedly on some subject. Are not his breaths short and deep?

PUPIL. Yes.

MASTER. Very well, now come with me to a concert. Mr. —— is singing Mendelssohn's "I'm a Roamer." Is not his breathing like that of the speaker, also short and deep?

PUPIL. Yes.

MASTER. Next observe the breathing of the athlete when running, jumping, or otherwise exerting himself. Finally, take a short, quick walk up hill yourself, and notice that both you and the athlete breathe quickly and deeply. From these observations you see that breathing when in a state of repose, or when one is not excited, differs from the breathing employed while exercising or labouring under emotion. These breathing lessons are given to prepare you for singing and speaking, which are physical and emotional exercises. As emotion increases or exercise grows more vigorous, breathing becomes deeper, fuller, and more rapid. The following exercises are given to produce and develop an outward movement of the lower ribs.

Exercise No. I.

Place one hand on the upper part of the chest, the other on the side, directly above the waist line, and without allowing the chest to rise, take six quick, short breaths, expiring after the last one in six short, quick, expiratory puffs.

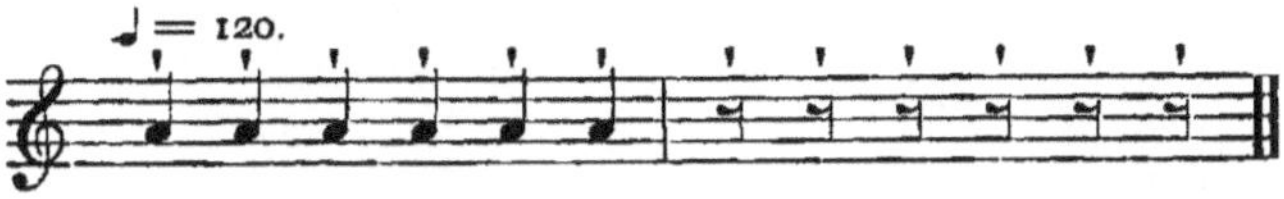

Inspiration. Expiration.

As soon as the outward movement of the ribs is strongly and sharply defined, you may begin Exercise No. II. as follows.

Exercise No. II.

After an ordinary inspiration, and while holding your breath, begin to draw in the abdomen and expand the ribs at the sides. These muscular acts are the same as the inspiratory movements, and are intended to increase and strengthen them.

You should practise exercises Nos. I. and II. until your lateral expansion has increased at least two inches before directing your thoughts to the other parts of inspiration. When this is accomplished you will have begun a development of the lower part of the chest, and this will continue with the increase of its other parts, until eventually you will have a lateral expansion of from four to five inches. This measurement indicates the expansion from fullest expiration to fullest inspiration.

LESSON III.

IN BREATHING.—THE BACKWARD EXPANSION.

MASTER. Did you ever, during exercise of any kind, notice a backward movement of the ribs?

PUPIL. No; at least, not until after my attention had been directed to it in the first lesson. I did not then know that they could move backward.

MASTER. If you will exercise violently for a few minutes until respiration becomes heavy and rapid, then place a hand upon your back, you will notice a very well-defined backward motion of the ribs. In order to feel this expansion the clothes must be loose, especially if corsets or other close-fitting garments have been habitually worn.

The deep breathing which occurs during exercise is called extraordinary breathing. During the most vigorous movements of extraordinary breathing, one may observe all the acts of ordinary breathing. You should carefully note all the movements taking place during gymnastic or other vigorous exercises, and *cultivate most those which are not strong in ordinary breathing.* The backward expansion, as you have observed, is one of your weak points; in fact, your lower ribs did not swing backward at all during ordinary inspiration.

PUPIL. Yes, I see. But why should there be weak places in one's breathing?

MASTER. Ah! Your question opens up a field of inquiry extending far beyond the scope of a lesson or two on breathing; but a general answer may give you a little help, and perhaps encourage personal observations and investigations which, properly directed and pursued, will lead to a full and satisfactory answer. *Whenever, on account of unwise dressing or from any other cause, the muscles are not sufficiently used, they become weak.* This fact calls attention to one of the principal reasons why vocalists so often make little or no progress in their studies. Even when they have discovered both a weakness and its cause, they endeavour to overcome the weakness without first removing the cause. This is a physical impossibility. If weakness or inactivity of muscle is due to dress, change your style of dress and give the imprisoned muscles freedom. In short, whatever be the cause it must be removed. You will then find that your ribs move backward, and that this backward swing is but a continuation of the lateral motion, which will be increased by the practice of the exercises given in the first lesson. In the development of the backward swing of the ribs, as in other exercises, the thoughts must be directed to the particular act desired. Do not allow the upper part of the chest to move very much in your first efforts to obtain a lateral, backward, or forward movement of the lower walls of the chest.

In order to procure a backward movement of the

ribs, bend the upper part of the body forward, and down as far as possible, next draw in the abdomen and take a short, quick, and deep breath, at the same time endeavouring to force the ribs out at the back. Assure yourself that the action of the abdomen and ribs at the back are those required by placing a hand on each of those places when inspiring the second time. These exercises should be practised until the movements become habitual in either the bent or the upright position.

LESSON IV.

In Breathing.—The Forward Expansion.

Master. In your first examination of the movements of the chest for inspiration you discovered only a very small forward movement of the ribs. Having found in Lesson III. that your ribs move backwards for an extraordinary inspiration, and having developed that movement, would you also expect a development of the forward movement at the same time?

Pupil. No, I do not see how there could be, at the same time, an expansion and development in both directions.

Master. If the attachment of the ribs to the spine at the back and to the breast-bone in front were on the same line, such a double movement would be impossible unless bone and cartilage were elastic. This, however, is not the case. The ribs hang out from the spine at such an angle that the attachment of one end of the rib to the spine is higher than the forward attachment of its other end to the breast-bone. In order to obtain a fairly correct idea on this point, suppose your body to be the spine, your arms two of the ribs, and your hands the breast-bone. "Place the back of the right hand in the palm of the left so that the fingers point in opposite directions, and the tips of the thumbs touch. Now let the arms form a circle and be held out from the body at about the angle of the sixth rib. This will bring the hands opposite the waist at a distance of about twelve inches. With the arms in this position, increase the distance between them laterally—that is, from elbow to elbow; at the same time raise them, but still preserve the circle." * After changing the position of your arms as directed, were the hands any further from your body?

PUPIL. Yes, they moved out from the body several inches.

MASTER. The exercise which you are to practise for the development of the forward expansion of your ribs is similar to that given for increasing their lateral movement; in fact, it is the amplification of the lateral and backward movements which produces the forward expansion.

In this exercise the breath is taken in by ten short inspiratory efforts, as indicated by the notes and staccato marks above them. The metronomical mark indicates the time to be given to the inspiration. Measures one, two, and three should be devoted to the lateral and backward movements, and measures four and five to the forward expansion.

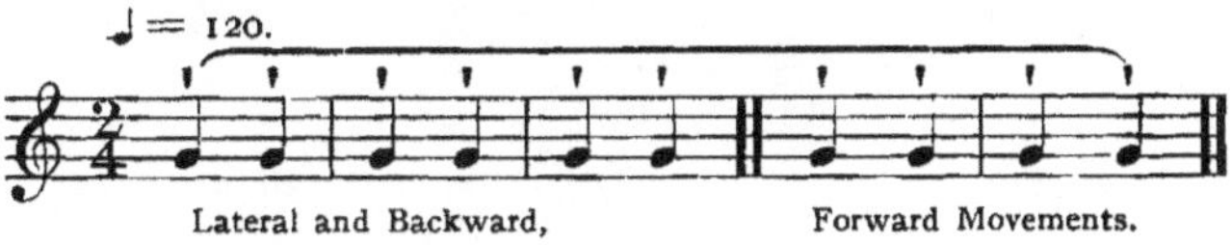

* From "Text Book on the Natural Use of the Voice," by George E. Thorp and William Nicholl.

When the chest is fully developed, women should have a lateral expansion of from four to five inches (men, on account of their greater stature, should have a little more) and a forward expansion of from one to one and a half inches, a backward expansion of three-quarters of an inch, and an upward movement of one inch. These are only approximate measurements for guiding you in your work. The development of the upper part of the chest is but a continuation of that begun in the lower part, and follows as a result of fuller inspiration. For its development the same short, deep breath is to be used, *followed, as it were, by a second breath higher in the chest.* To guide you in this practice, place one hand on your side just above the waist line, the other on the upper part of the chest. Take the short, deep inspiration as directed in previous lessons, stop a second, then continue with as full an expansion of the entire chest as possible. In this exercise give particular attention to those movements of inspiration by which the upper part of the chest is expanded.

LESSON V.

IN BREATHING.—THE UPWARD EXPANSION.

MASTER. When observing the movements of the book or ruler which you placed upon your chest as directed in the first lesson, you saw it move both out and up. The necessity for the upward movement and its development now claims your attention.

In the act of inspiration, does the air enter the lungs and force out the walls of the chest, or do you by muscular effort draw out the walls and so suck in the air?

PUPIL. Never having thought of inspiration in that way I cannot say at once; but let me think a moment. I do not see that force is being used to propel air into my lungs; I therefore conclude that it must, in some way, be drawn in by the expansions of the chest walls.

MASTER. You are right. "The lungs," says Huxley, "are a kind of suction pump." The principle upon which they are inflated and afterward exhausted of air is the same as that upon which the syringe is worked. If you perform the following experiment with an ordinary glass syringe, you will learn how the air is taken into the lungs. After placing the open end of the syringe in water, draw out its handle. This act tends to create a vacuum in the syringe, which, however, is prevented by the water being drawn up through the open tube, and the space within is filled with water. In the case of the lungs, the lateral, backward, forward, and upward movements of the ribs tend in the same way to create a vacuum, but the air is drawn in through the nose, or mouth, and the windpipe, which are permanently open, and fills the lungs.

Two more questions must be considered before you take up the exercises for the development of the upward movement of the chest.

First, do you know the boundaries of the lungs? The second, do you know whether an upward movement of the collar-bone is necessary in order to fully inflate the lungs?

PUPIL. No, I do not think I can answer those questions.

The floor or base of the lungs rests upon the convex surface of the diaphragm, a cone-shaped muscle which separates the trunk of the body into two parts. This division begins at the end of the breast-bone and extends a little lower down at the sides and back. The breast-bone, ribs, and backbone form the boundaries of the front, side, and back of the lungs. At the top they extend upwards into the neck from $1\frac{1}{4}$ to $1\frac{3}{4}$ inches above the first ribs. If you mark these boundary lines on your body, you will find that the lungs occupy a much smaller part of the trunk than you supposed. In fact, they fill less than half of it.

On account of imperfect movements of the walls of the chest, the upper part of the lungs is not regularly used in breathing. The angle at which the ribs hang out from the spine, makes that part of the lung cavity which extends upward into the root of the neck very small. The lungs, windpipe, great blood-vessels, &c., fill the space, so that, in the usual low position of the upper part of the chest, this part of the lungs can receive very little air. The cartilaginous connection between the upper ribs and the breast-bone is very short, and since the cartilages have very little or no power of expansion, the increase in the chest must be made by an upward and outward movement of the chest walls at this place.

LESSON VI.

IN BREATHING.—THE UPWARD MOVEMENT OF THE CHEST, CONTINUED.

MASTER. From your study of inspiration, up to this point, can you tell what act gives the greatest increase in the size of the chest, and consequently in the lung capacity?

PUPIL. Yes; the greatest increase is the result of a change in the position of the walls; that is, the lateral, backward, upward, and forward movements which I have already noticed, not a stretching of the chest walls as I formerly thought.

MASTER. Do the collar-bones always rise with the elevation of the chest?

PUPIL. The inner ends rise, but the outer ends may or may not rise. It depends upon whether I raise my shoulders when I breathe.

MASTER. The first exercise for the raising and expansion of the upper part of the chest is a muscular act, which is to be practised independent of respiration. After a normal inspiration, and while holding the breath, *draw in the abdomen and diminish the girth of the body at the waist line, at the same time raise the upper part of the chest.* When, by means of this muscular exercise, you can raise your chest an inch or so, begin to practise it during respiration, raising the chest for inspiration and allowing it to fall for expiration.

Through practice, this movement will become habitual, then all parts of inspiration must be undertaken with one breath, and be cultivated until this method of inspiring is natural. In order to obtain the greatest possible working capacity of the lungs, there still remains a point of great importance. After a normal expiration there is a large quantity of air left in the lungs. A part of this air is called "residual air," and cannot be expelled, but the remainder, called "supplementary air," you can learn to force out by practising the following exercise. After ordinary expiration contract the lower ribs as much as possible, and bring the shoulders as far forward as possible, so as to let the upper part of the chest fall in, and at the same time bend the upper part of the body forward. In this way a large quantity of supplementary air will be expelled which would otherwise have remained in the lungs. Like the inspiratory exercise, this should be practised daily. Having carefully studied all these lessons, and practised the exercises as directed, you should find that the difference between full expiration and full inspiration is approximately as follows:

Lateral expansion, four inches.

Forward and backward expansion, one and a half inches.

Elevation of chest, one inch.

Increase between first and ninth rib, one inch.
Circular expansion, four inches.
Below the nipple line, six inches.

This method of inspiration gives breath adequate to all demands upon the voice; it also plays an important part, as you will see, in the power and quality of the voice.

LESSON VII.

POWER.

MASTER. All those who wish to develop the voice should know that its power and quality depend to a large extent upon the amount of air in the lungs, it's degree of density, and its proximity to the vocal organs. In order to demonstrate this, I ask you to select for resonators * two or more prune jars differing in size, the largest one containing about a pint. Next put a tuning fork into vibration, and with its flat side up, pass it over the open end of each jar, beginning with the smallest, and state what effect is produced on the sound of the fork.

PUPIL. When I held the fork in my hand away from the jars it had very little sound, but when I held it above the smallest one the sound was louder, and it increased in power as I held it above the larger jar.

MASTER. From these observations do you think that a resonance chamber could be increased indefinitely, and still continue to reinforce the sound?

---

* For full information on Resonators see chap. 16 in "Text Book on the Natural Use of the Voice," by George E. Thorp and William Nicholl. Published by Robert Cocks and Co., 6, New Burlington-street, London, W.

PUPIL. I should think so, had not experience taught me that such is not the case.

MASTER. What observations have you made regarding this point?

PUPIL. I have noticed that at sea, or on extensive plains, the most lusty shout seems a thin, small sound, which is quickly lost in space; also, that in a valley surrounded by precipitous cliffs or mountains the voice (or its echo) sounds much louder than at sea. Again, I have heard the voice of a street singer grow suddenly stronger when he entered a street with tall houses on both sides.

MASTER. From your observations and the experiment with fork and bottle, have you drawn any conclusions helpful to you in your work?

PUPIL. Yes, I think the voice attains its maximum power when used in a room of proper dimensions. In experimenting with the fork I found that its sound was greater with each increase in the size of the bottle up to a certain point, beyond that size the fork's sound began to diminish. In the case of the voice when used in an unlimited space there was very little tone, as the area became limited the tone grew stronger until the proper dimensions were found. A greater diminution of the air space either causes the voice to sound smaller or destroys its quality.

MASTER. Your observations are very interesting, but have you not noticed that the experiment with fork and bottle was made, first with a small bottle which had only a little air space, then with larger bottles having more space, while the sounds of the voice, you say, increased in power as the *space grew less.*

PUPIL. Yes, that seeming discrepancy confronted me when trying the fork-and-bottle experiment. After a moment's thought, however, it appeared quite clear. Having larger bottles beside me when I tried the experiment with the fork, I also held it above them, and found that, exceeding a certain sized bottle, the sound of the fork grew less until no reinforcement could be heard.

Another incident, also bearing upon this point, came under my observation a few days since. A child and a kitten were playing together upon the floor; inadvertently the child trod upon the kitten's foot, causing it to utter a howl of pain. The howl, which was not loud at first, rapidly developed into a very strong cry. The child, pleased, no doubt, with this sound, at once imitated it. In both these cases, when the sound was soft the mouth was nearly closed, when the sound became strong the mouth was wide open.* I then made a few experiments, using the utmost care not to increase the fundamental tone while gradually opening the mouth, and found the result to be the same as when holding the fork above the bottles, the sound increased with enlarged space.

MASTER. From these experiments and your observations, has it occurred to you that similar principles are

---

* The separation of the teeth, noticed by the pupil in these instances, did not increase the power of the sound. The increase

involved in the use of other air chambers found in the body?

PUPIL. Yes, that is now clear to me. Formerly I noticed great variations in the power and quality of voices, and supposing them to be natural gave them no thought.

MASTER. It is true that voices differ naturally just as features do; but it is also true that in the majority of cases we do not hear the natural power and quality of the voice, because some of the air chambers in the body, which serve to increase the power of the voice, are not kept so fully open as they should be. There is no doubt that, in the natural growth of the body, each organ and chamber should attain those dimensions necessary for the symmetry of the structure as a whole, and adequate for the various functions to be performed. One of these functions, as we now know, is the reinforcement of sound.

LESSON VIII.

BREATH CONTROL.

MASTER. Most students think that a full expiration exhausts the air in the lungs. Do you think the same?

PUPIL. I did, but in Lesson VI. I learned that, after a normal expiration, a large amount of air still remains in the lungs.

MASTER. Why does not the residual air leave the lungs during the act of expiration?

PUPIL. I do not know.

MASTER. Again the ordinary glass syringe used in a previous experiment may serve to illustrate this point. The water is forced out of the syringe by pushing in the handle, and thus diminishing the space within the tube which contains the water. In this case it is possible to force out all the water by completely closing the space in the tube, but the chest walls cannot be brought closely enough together to fully close the cavity within them; therefore, all the air cannot be driven out, even though the tube through which it passes is wide open. From these observations, which agents do you think control the act of respiration?

PUPIL. To me it appears that those muscles which increase and diminish the size of the chest cavity must govern the respiratory act.

MASTER. While the body and mind are in a state of repose that is true; but when respiration becomes extraordinary, that is, active instead of passive, there comes into use a set of organs not used before, and evidently designed for the demands now made upon them. For example, when we cough the breath is checked for a moment, then suddenly released, and leaves the throat with a violent explosive sound, does it not?

PUPIL. Yes.

MASTER. If the tube through which the breath passed were permanently open, could there have been an explosive sound?

PUPIL. I should think not.

MASTER. You think then that it is possible to close the tube at some point?

PUPIL. Yes.

MASTER. Cough vigorously and try to locate the point where the tube closes.

PUPIL. I think the breath is stopped within the larynx (Adam's apple).

MASTER. That is right, and the name of the organs which prevent the exit of the air is the *False Vocal Chords*. Of these you will learn more in subsequent lessons. Now notice. Coughing is a strong physical effort, for which the breath is always momentarily stopped by the False Vocal Chords. Now I will ask you to lift a heavy weight and hold it out for a moment at arm's length. Did you exhale while holding the weight?

PUPIL. No.

MASTER. What prevented the air from leaving the lungs?

PUPIL. I felt the same closure at the larynx as before; therefore, I suppose, the False Vocal Chords closed when I began to lift, and remained closed until effort ceased.

MASTER. Again lift the weight, and hold it out as before and note the movement of those muscles about the walls of the lower part of the chest. Do they increase or diminish the size of the lower part of the chest?

PUPIL. They contract and diminish the girth of the body at that point.

MASTER. Here again notice, lifting is a physical act, for which the breath is held in check by the False Vocal Chords.* For both these physical acts of coughing and lifting, the breath was forced upward and stopped. This resistance to the upward pressure of the breath causes the air in the lungs to become compressed. This compression takes place in all vigorous efforts.

---

* See chapter on expiration in "Text Book on the Natural Use of the Voice." By George E. Thorp and William Nicholl.

LESSON IX.

Breath Control.

Master. In the last lesson you learned that the breath must be compressed for all vigorous physical effort. In this lesson you will learn that the same is true in singing. Moreover, in singing you must maintain the compression during the gradual emission of the air required to set the vocal organs into vibration, and when this has been accomplished you will have acquired breath control.

For your first exercise take a full breath, hold it a moment, and while doing so draw in the abdomen and lower ribs a little. Having in this way compressed the air, allow it to escape suddenly, making an explosive breath sound in which the vowel sound of "U" (as in the word "utter") is heard. While the breath escapes, keep the compression unaltered by gradually diminishing the size of the lower part of the chest. At first you should judge of the regularity of the outward flowing breath by the continuity of the breathy "Uh" sound. When this sound can be maintained with a steady pressure and an even power, diminish the sound as much as possible. Continue to practice this exercise without tone, until you can regulate the emission, and make your breath last at least thirty seconds.

Both power and quality of the voice are altered by varying the compression of the air in the lungs. This fact is of great importance, and I wish you to become thoroughly conversant with it. Therefore, I call your attention to two experiments which demonstrate it.

EXPERIMENT NO. I.

Place an electric bell within a glass jar, then seal the jar and exhaust the air by means of an air pump. Next set the bell ringing, it produces no sound because there is no air in the jar to be set into vibration. By means of a small tube allow the air to enter the jar very slowly, and the sound which becomes audible with the first entry of air steadily grows louder until the jar is full. The density of the air within is now the same as that outside the jar and the tone has reached its normal power. By means of a second pump, more air is forced into the jar, and the sound of the bell continues to increase until no more air can be introduced.

It is impossible for most students of singing to perform this experiment, as they have not the necessary apparatus at hand; therefore I give the second experiment, equally good and much more simple, which all can perform.

Probably you know that heat expands the air, if, therefore, you heat a jar, the air within is expanded, and if one end of the jar is open part of the air will be expelled, which is equivalent to pumping some of it out.

EXPERIMENT NO. II.

For this experiment select several glass jars open at one end, and heat them so that the air within registers approximately 200°, 170°, 140°, 110°, 80° Fahr. The sixth jar should not be heated. Now sound a tuning fork and hold it, with its flat side up, over each jar in the order given. How is the sound of the fork affected ?

PUPIL. When I held it above the first jar, which was the hottest, there was no alteration in the tone; above the second, in which the air was colder, I could detect a very slight increase in the power of the sound; and over each succeeding jar, having a lower temperature, there was a further increase in the power of the sound.

MASTER. Perhaps you do not see how all this applies to your voice.

PUPIL. I must confess that I do not, because I can neither pump air into my lungs after inspiration, nor make the imprisoned air colder.

MASTER. Very true; but after filling your lungs you can diminish the air space within them, and in that way compress the air.

The air-gun used by children as a toy will help you to understand how air can be compressed, and at the same time demonstrate how sound is increased when it is made in compressed air. Draw out the handle of the gun and the barrel will be filled with air. Now put a cork into the end so as to prevent the air from escaping when the handle is pressed in. We will suppose that the barrel of the gun is a foot long and that you push the handle in four inches. What has become of the air that was in that four-inch space?

PUPIL. It was pressed forward into the first eight inches of the tube.

MASTER. Was not that part of the tube full before?

PUPIL. Yes, but I suppose that it was not packed full.

MASTER. I like your term "packed full," as it expresses more to a student than compressed. Let us now notice how this packed air affects sound. Press the cork lightly into the end of the gun and push in the handle. The cork is quickly forced from the gun and an explosive sound, low in pitch, and having but little power, is produced. Again, place the cork in the gun, but more firmly. This time more force is required to expel it, and the tone is both stronger and higher in pitch.

So long as the cork continues to present greater resistance the air must be more compressed to blow it out, and the accompanying sound will become both stronger and higher in pitch.

As stated above, the air taken into the lungs can, by the elasticity of the lungs themselves and the contraction of the walls surrounding them, be pressed into a much smaller space than it occupies when first inspired. According to Dr. Hutchinson, the pressure thus brought to bear upon the inspired air may reach 1000lb. However this may be, if you take a full breath, and hold it either at the lips or in the throat, and at the same time try to expel it from the lungs, you will realise that a very great pressure is brought to bear upon it.

It is said that Rubini, exerting himself for a high tone, pressed his breath upwards with such force that his collar-bone was broken.

From these facts and experiments you have learned that sound in general increases with increasing density, or compression of the air. You have also learned to compress, or make more dense, the air in your lungs, and have observed that as a consequence of that compression your voice has increased in power.

Continual practice of the exercise given at the beginning of this lesson for breath compression and breath control will perfect you in both these respects, and at the same time increase the power of your voice and enrich its quality.

LESSON X.

BREATH CONTROL.

MASTER. It is comparatively easy to control one's breath when one is not making sound, but when the breath is employed to produce tone its control becomes much more difficult. I have met a few students who managed their breath well from the beginning, but the majority do not, and this is to them a very important lesson.

Before beginning it let me relate an incident which shows that one does not always hear his voice as others hear it, and also that one may be totally unaware of his most conspicuous fault. A lady, singing for the first time to her master, was asked, "How does your voice sound to you?" In reply she said, "The quality appears good, but the tone is not strong enough." From this answer it was evident that she had never heard her own voice as a casual listener would hear it; therefore she was told that her first lessons would be devoted to analysing her present tone, to discover if the quality really were good as she thought. This lesson and the next were devoted to a study of her old production. When she returned a third time it was to announce her intention to discontinue lessons, saying that her voice was growing breathy, and that she always understood that breath in the tone would eventually destroy the voice for singing purposes. Her master of course said that he could not prevent her from going, but before leaving he should like to ask her a question. To this she consented, and he asked, "In the two lessons which you have taken, what have I requested you to do?" After a moment's thought she said as though to herself, "Yes, it is true; you have asked me to do nothing but listen." This lady had learned to hear in her voice that which all her friends had heard, but of which she herself was up to that time wholly unconscious.

Study your voice and listen to it very carefully before beginning to develop it, because the breath element, from which very few voices are free, is not always strong enough to attract your attention. This is specially so in the robust sounds of the voice. If your tones are breathy you will probably discover it in singing the following exercises.

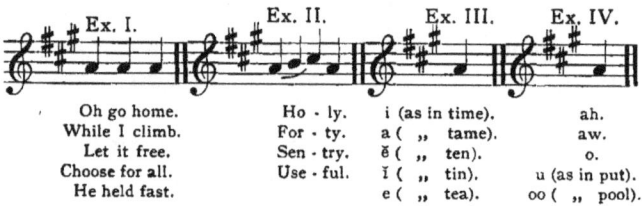

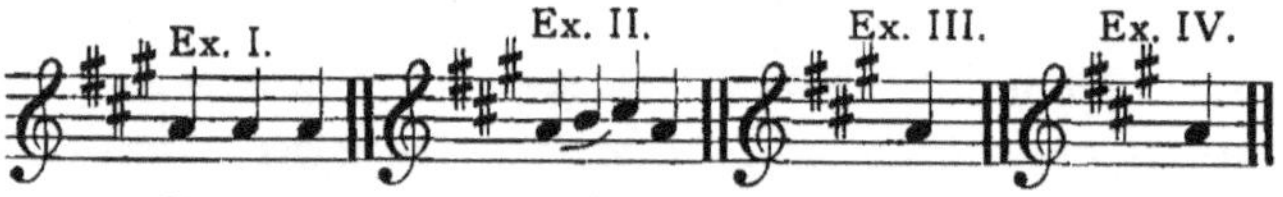

Ex. I.	Ex. II.	Ex. III.	Ex. IV.
Oh go home.	Ho - ly.	i (as in time).	ah.
While I climb.	For - ty.	a („ tame).	aw.
Let it free.	Sen - try.	ĕ („ ten).	o.
Choose for all.	Use - ful.	ĭ („ tin).	u (as in put).
He held fast.		e („ tea).	oo („ pool).

Did you hear breathy tones in any of these exercises?

PUPIL. I am not perfectly clear as to what you mean by a "breathy tone."

MASTER. Have you ever heard the sound of the flute-player's breath upon his instrument as he plays?

PUPIL. Oh, yes, very often; but does one hear such sounds in the voice?

MASTER. Not so strong as a rule, but very few even of our best vocalists are without it on some words. In Lesson IX. you learned to control your breath without tone. You may use the same exercise again, but in this instance the out-going breath must be vocalised.

Sing the exercise now, and use "uh" as the vocal sound. Was the tone pure?

PUPIL. No, I heard both tone and breath.

MASTER. Masters in their efforts to overcome the breathy sound in the voice have used such expressions as "drink in the tone," "sing as though you were yawning," "sing in," "draw in your breath," "drink in your voice," "sing into your head," or "sing into your chest," and no doubt many others, all of which are based upon sensations which arise from the following fact. The instant that the out-going breath is interrupted or partly checked, it begins to accumulate and becomes condensed, expanding the chamber in which it is confined. The sensation arising from this opposition to the outward flow of the breath, and at the same time from the outward expansion of the walls of the trachea and chest, is similar to the sensation caused by the expansion of those parts for inspiration.

While these expressions do not accurately describe the physical movements taking place, they usually lead the student to correct his fault, and on this account they must not be wholly condemned.

Practise the following exercise to get rid of the breathy sound.

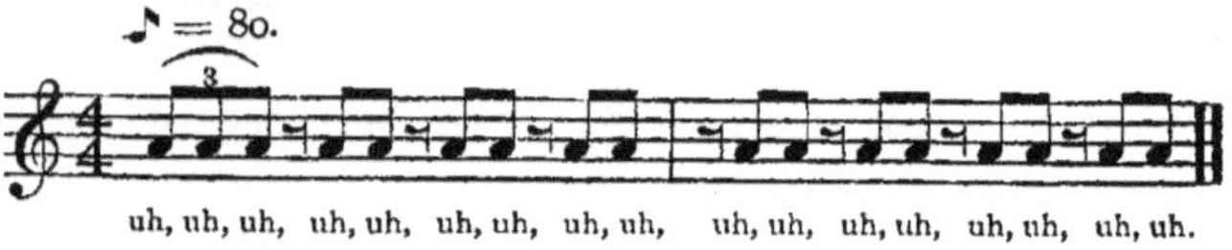

CAUTIONS.

1. In this exercise, although all the sounds are to be taken short at first, there should be no thought of singing the notes staccato.

2. Sing at natural power, that is, mezzo forte.

3. Sing in exact metronomical time.

4. Sing all the tones as short as possible.

5. Listen for breathy tones, and if you detect any try to avoid them.

6. Make each tone by an action in the throat, like the one made when you coughed, *not by an action of the ribs.*

7. Do not allow the ribs to move until after the tone is made.

8. Do not breathe before the end of the exercise.

Practise this exercise, observing these cautions, until the short tones are pure, then prolong the sound of each tone until you can hold a pure tone as long as you formerly held the breathy sound without tone.

When you practise this exercise, what position does your chest assume?

PUPIL. It rises as high as possible.

MASTER. Does this high position of your chest affect the tones of your voice?

PUPIL. I do not know, but I think it does.

MASTER. There is a prejudice against the elevation of the chest for singing or speaking. Some masters go so far as to condemn the least movement of the upper ribs. Your next lesson will be devoted to settling that question, but meanwhile let your chest rise.

LESSON XI.

Breath Control.

It is essential that students of singing should know that altering the size, shape, and position of the various organs employed in tone production varies both power and quality of the voice. Most students do not know this, or if they do, they fail to make use of their knowledge in singing. You have already learned, in Lesson VII., how varying the size of the air chamber alters the tone, and now a few examples are given to show that an air chamber, when in proper proximity to a sound, reinforces that sound. Observe first, that the sound of the locomotive whistle grows louder and more shrill as the train approaches the mouth of a tunnel; second, the music of a band grows suddenly louder as the band passes close to the open door of a large hall; third, that the sound of a tuning fork, when put into vibration and held just above an open jar, is much stronger than when removed two or three inches from it; and, lastly, the ordinary speaking trumpet used to increase the power of the human voice can only do so when the trumpet is placed close to or upon the mouth of the speaker.

Many more examples might be given, but those mentioned represent a large enough variety of reinforced sounds to show that the principle is a general one. The tone-producing agent and the resonance chamber must be brought into close proximity to increase the intrinsic tone. The question now arises, how does this apply to the voice?

The intrinsic tone of the vocal chords is very small, the singing tone of the voice is strong; therefore, the singing tone is a reinforced sound. The intrinsic tone is produced in an air chamber which communicates with several other larger chambers, all of which are employed in increasing the power of the intrinsic tone. The degree of reinforcement obtained from these chambers depends upon their distance from the vocal organs. You have learned that the greatest air chamber in the body (the thoracic cavity which contains the lungs) is raised, in extraordinary respiration, and while singing the exercise given in Lesson X. you found that you raised your chest as much as possible. At this time I wish you to observe that that act diminishes the distance between the chest and the vocal chords, an inch or more. You have also found that the vocal organs, on account of their position and the construction of the tube in which they are placed, can be brought into closer relation to the chest cavity. In fact, these organs fall from three-quarters of an inch to an inch and a quarter for the production of good tones, and the result is a marked increase in the power of the tone. Thus you see that the prejudice which would not allow the chest to be raised for singing or speaking would, if indulged in, prevent the voice from attaining its natural or full degree of power.

In the last lesson you learned to produce a continuous tone at one pitch without an escape of breath; you must next learn to change the pitch and preserve a pure tone, first at a uniform power, then varying from loud to soft and *vice versa*. For this purpose practise the following exercises with the vowels, o, i, a, ah, aw, u (as in the word "but"), and oo (as in "pool").

Practise first at natural power and with uniform quality.

Practise next beginning each exercise *p* and *cres.*

Practise lastly beginning each exercise *f* and *dim.*

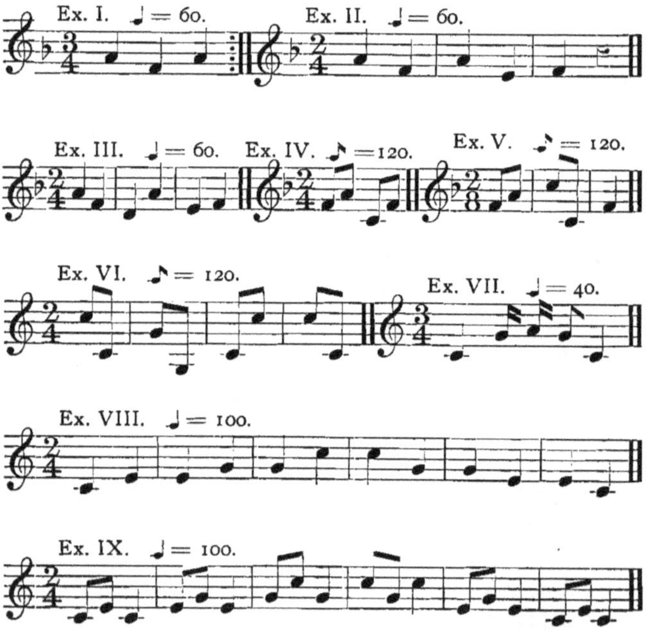

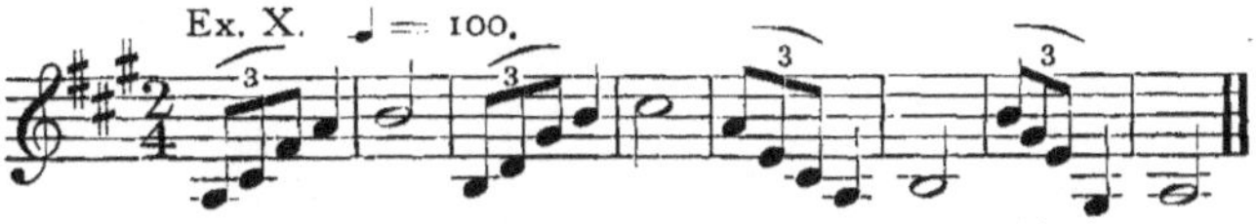

Soprano and Tenor Voices sing these Exercises a minor third higher.

These exercises are varied enough to cover the ground of change of pitch. They should be practised first legato, then staccato. This latter form of singing requires an action of the respiratory muscles somewhat unlike those used in legato singing. When you produce a succession of short, quick sounds, called staccato, the false vocal chords should take and remain in the position they have when you sing a continuous sound. These tones are the result of an abrupt and vigorous inward movement of the ribs. You will get a very good idea of those movements if you fix a whistle upon the end of a pair of hand-bellows, and, after filling the bellows with air, press upon the handles so as to make four separate or disconnected sounds in a second. When you sing staccato you do not completely close the air passage from the lungs, hence the necessity for the spasmodic thoracic efforts. The sudden contraction of the walls produces a sound, and the equally abrupt relaxation causes the tone to cease. *Under these circumstances*—that is, the open condition of the tube and the spasmodic actions of the ribs—*there cannot be a continuous compression of the air in the lungs, and the voice, when singing staccato, can never be used at its full power.*

LESSON XII.

Breath Control.

Now that you have learned to control your breath, both with and without tone, while singing vowel sounds at a fixed pitch or in a melody, and to manage the ribs for staccato singing, you must also learn to control your breath while forming and using consonants with the vowels. You will see the importance of this requirement if you pronounce the following words and notice the amount of escaping breath in each: "push," "flash," "thrust," "crust," "kin," "choice," "cease," "show," "James," and "switch." The redundancy of breath in these words is due to the habit of forming the consonants with breath from the lungs and giving them undue prominence. For example, place the hand upon your chest while pronouncing vigorously, but not aloud, the following letters, and notice that the chest falls with each: p, f, t, c, and k.

The breath in the lungs should be used for tone production, and the air in the mouth for articulation.

The voice organs, which are set into vibration by the breath from the lungs, and the articulating organs, which employ the air in the mouth in forming the sounds of the letters, are entirely independent of each other. Moreover, they are situated in separate chambers. Although these facts indicate that our present task is an easy one; it is not so, and requires close attention and long application before it is accomplished. When you pronounce the words "*pound*" and "*flow,*" giving the first letter in each word a strong accent, do either your lips or cheeks expand with compressed air?

PUPIL. Yes, both lips and cheeks are inflated.

MASTER. Place your hand on the upper part of your chest and pronounce in a loud whisper the words "pound" and "flow." Did the chest fall with the explosion of the compressed air in your cheeks?

PUPIL. Oh, yes, the chest fell quickly at first, then slowly until I had finished the word.

MASTER. Now pronounce in the same way the first letter in each word, and see if the chest falls as it did before.

PUPIL. Yes, the movements were the same in kind, but somewhat less in extent.

MASTER. This shows that the door (False Vocal Chords) separating the air chamber in the chest from the chambers above in the pharynx, mouth, and head, is open, and that you not only inflated the lips and cheeks with breath from your lungs, but also used that breath to prolong the sound of the consonants. As I have already said, when you are making the consonants, this door, which controls the imprisoned breath, should never be opened unless the breath is required to produce sound.

PUPIL. But can I make the consonants strong enough to be heard if I close that passage?

MASTER. Yes, there is sufficient air in your mouth to give to each consonant as much power as it can have.

PUPIL. When I sing such words as "only," "holy," "going," &c., the consonants following the vowels must be made while I am making tone; can I avoid using the air from the lungs in forming them?

MASTER. There are a few consonants, and those you have mentioned are among them, which, like the vowels, are known by the quality of their sound, that is, the *vocal* sound which these letters have. Those consonants require no breath. Neither their position nor action produces or is accompanied by a hissing or explosive sound. The explosive "p," the blowing "f," and the hissing "s" are examples of consonants on which breath is wasted. In order to gain breath control when forming these and similar letters, you must be able to make them distinctly and with sufficient power *while holding your breath.* What is the first thing you do when you say "p" as in the word "post?"

PUPIL. I press my lips together.

MASTER. We call that act taking the position for the consonant. What do you do next?

PUPIL. I separate the lips.

MASTER. This we call the action of the letter.

Accompanying the separation of the lips what occurred?

PUPIL. There was an explosive sound.

MASTER. What caused the explosion?

PUPIL. The sudden release of the compressed air in my mouth.

MASTER. If the explosive sound is breathy and can be prolonged two or more seconds, it is certain that breath is escaping from the lungs. In this case you must hold your breath and say the letter again When properly made, the explosive sound will resemble that made when a cork is drawn from an empty bottle. When you have learned to pronounce "p" correctly, practise the phonetic sounds of the following letters until no breath escapes from the lungs while forming them.

Breath Consonants, P, Wh, F, Th (thin), S, T, Sh, H (high), and K.

Voice Consonants, B, W, V, Th (then), Z, D, L, R, and G.

During the practice of all these letters, hold one hand on your chest to assist in detecting an escape of breath from the lungs. A falling of the chest indicates the loss of breath. When you can form these letters quickly and powerfully as directed, it is time to join them to tone. In either speaking or singing the words, the vocal sound and the articulate sound are never produced simultaneously. In order to maintain an independent action of the different sets of muscles, as well as to obtain the proper use of the breath in the lungs and the air in the mouth, you must, at first, increase the natural interval of time between the consonants and the vowel sounds. In the following exercises, the separation is indicated in the music.

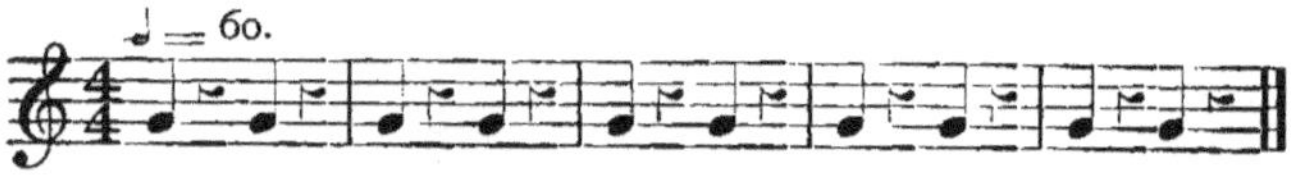

P - ah,	P - aw,	P - oh,	P - u,*	P - oo.†
F - ah,	F - aw,	F - oh,	F - u,	F - oo.
Th- ah,‡	Th- aw,	Th- oh,	Th- u,	Th- oo.
S - ah,	S - aw,	S - oh,	S - u,	S - oo.
Sh- ah,	Sh- aw,	Sh- oh,	Sh- u,	Sh- oo.
Ch- ah,	Ch- aw,	Ch- oh,	Ch- u,	Ch- oo.
J - ah,	J - aw,	J - oh,	J - u,	J - oo.
G§- ah,	G - aw,	G - oh,	G - u,	G - oo.

The position, action, and sound of the consonant precedes and is separated from the vowel sound in this exercise. In your next exercise the vowel precedes the consonant, otherwise these exercises are alike.

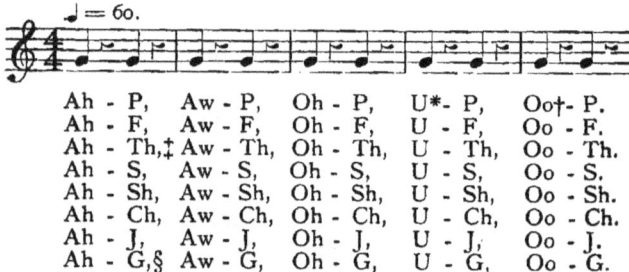

Ah - P,	Aw - P,	Oh - P,	U*- P,	Oo†- P.
Ah - F,	Aw - F,	Oh - F,	U - F,	Oo - F.
Ah - Th,‡	Aw - Th,	Oh - Th,	U - Th,	Oo - Th.
Ah - S,	Aw - S,	Oh - S,	U - S,	Oo - S.
Ah - Sh,	Aw - Sh,	Oh - Sh,	U - Sh,	Oo - Sh.
Ah - Ch,	Aw - Ch,	Oh - Ch,	U - Ch,	Oo - Ch.
Ah - J,	Aw - J,	Oh - J,	U - J,	Oo - J.
Ah - G,§	Aw - G,	Oh - G,	U - G,	Oo - G.

Following the lip vowels in these exercises come he tongue vowels, after the practice of which you

* U (as in the word pull). † Oo (as in the word pool).
‡ Th (as in the word thin). § G (as in gun).

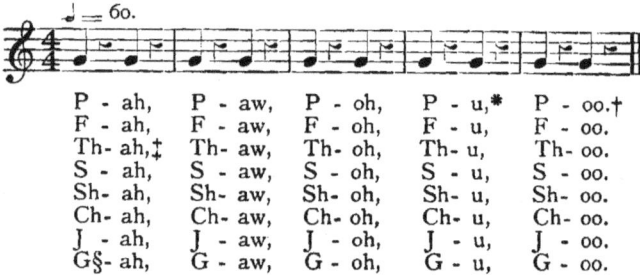

must diminish the interval between vowel and consonant until there is no appreciable pause between them.

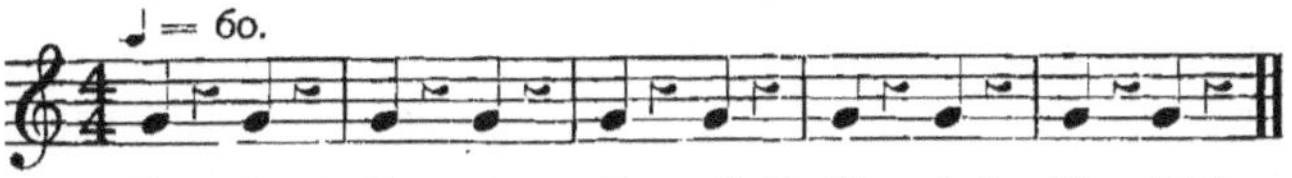

P - I,	P - A,	P - E,*	P - I,†	P - E.‡
F - I,	F - A,	F - E,	F - I,	F - E.
Th - I,§	Th - A,	Th - E,	Th - I,	Th - E.
S - I,	S - A,	S - E,	S - I,	S - E.
Sh - I,	Sh - A,	Sh - E,	Sh - I,	Sh - E.
Ch - I,	Ch - A,	Ch - E,	Ch - I,	Ch - E.
J - I,	J - A,	J - E,	J - I,	J - E.
G‖ - I,	G - A,	G - E,	G - I,	G - E.

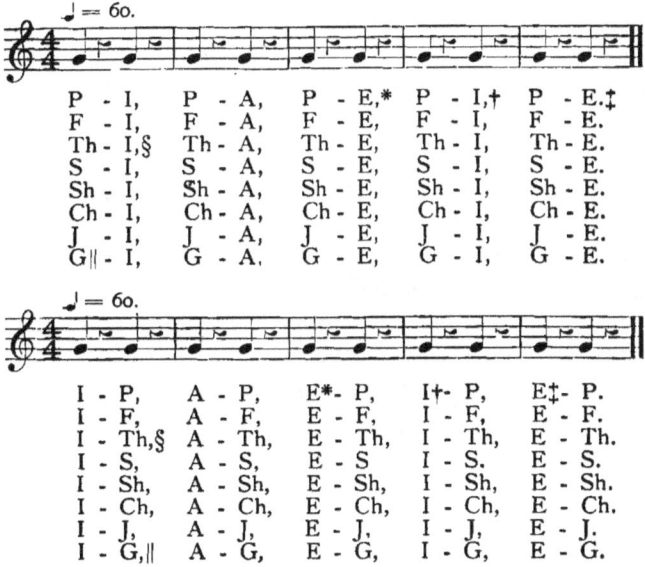

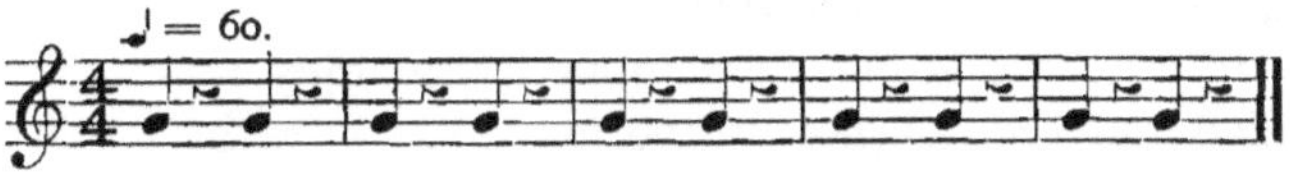

I - P,	A - P,	E* - P,	I† - P,	E‡ - P.
I - F,	A - F,	E - F,	I - F,	E - F.
I - Th,§	A - Th,	E - Th,	I - Th,	E - Th.
I - S,	A - S,	E - S	I - S.	E - S.
I - Sh,	A - Sh,	E - Sh,	I - Sh,	E - Sh.
I - Ch,	A - Ch,	E - Ch,	I - Ch,	E - Ch.
I - J,	A - J,	E - J,	I - J,	E - J.
I - G,‖	A - G,	E - G,	I - G,	E - G.

With the exception of "G" and "J" all the consonants in these exercises are breath consonants, that is, letters having no vocal sound in them. Let us analyse the pronunciation of the vocal consonant "B" in "boy" and the breath consonant "P" in "poise," to find in what respect they are unlike. In the pronunciation of "p" we have first the compressed

---

* E (as in pen). † I (as in pin). ‡ E (as in pea).
§ Th (as in thin). ‖ G (as in gun).

position of the lips, next the compression of the air in the mouth, and lastly the separation of the lips accompanied with an explosive sound of the air in the mouth. For "b," the lips are pressed together as for "p," the air in the mouth is compressed, and a vocal sound low down in the throat is made. This sound continues during the explosive breath sound caused by the separation of the lips, and finally becomes the vowel "o" which follows in the word "boy." On account of the similarity between the vocal and breath consonants, the exercise already given will answer for both.

If your work has been done thoroughly, and you have mastered each of these lessons, you will be able to inspire and fill your lungs quickly, quietly, and without apparent effort. Moreover, you will be able to place, compress, and control your breath, thus making it equal to all demands.

THE END.

ROBERT COCKS & CO.'S MODERN METHODS.—No. 13.

TWENTY LESSONS

ON THE

DEVELOPMENT OF THE VOICE

FOR

SINGERS, SPEAKERS, AND TEACHERS.

BY

GEORGE E. THORP,

Lecturer on, and Teacher of, "Voice Production."

AUTHOR OF

"COLOUR AUDITION AND ITS RELATION TO VOICE PRODUCTION,"
"TWELVE LESSONS ON BREATHING AND BREATH CONTROL,"

AND CO-AUTHOR OF

"A TEXT-BOOK ON THE NATURAL USE OF THE VOICE."

This Series of Lessons is intended to give Singers, Teachers, Orators, Elocutionists, and Clergymen a Practical Knowledge of How to Strengthen and Develop the Voice.

PRICE 1/-

London:

ROBERT COCKS & CO.,

Music Publishers to H.M. the Queen and H.R.H. the Prince of Wales.

6, NEW BURLINGTON STREET, W.

Agents for the United States of America: EDWARD SCHUBERTH & CO., New York.

VOICE PRODUCTION.

A SIMPLE AND PRACTICAL METHOD

FOR THE

Cultivation of tone and improvement of the Singing Voice, together with a carefully graduated Series of Exercises suited to the progressive requirements of Students.

BY

EDWIN HOLLAND,

Professor of Singing at the Royal Academy of Music, Guildhall School, &c., &c.

A SPECIAL FEATURE

BEING THE

SEPARATE AND COMPREHENSIVE TREATMENT OF EACH VOICE,

WITH NUMEROUS ILLUSTRATIONS AND NOTES.

Cloth, 5/- *net.* COPYRIGHT. *Paper,* 4/- *net.*

In Six Parts, each Voice complete ... ... *each* 1/6 *net.*

LONDON:

ROBERT COCKS & CO.,

6. NEW BURLINGTON STREET, W

Music Publishers to H.M. the Queen and H.R.H. the Prince of Wales.

AGENTS FOR THE UNITED STATES OF AMERICA:

EDWARD SCHUBERTH & CO., New York.

"Daily Vocal Exercises"

BY

CIRO PINSUTI.

The object of these Exercises is to enable all who sing (with or without the aid of a master) to secure the development of the voice, by a regular daily practice of some of these useful Vocal Exercises. They are written by Signor Pinsuti as the result of over thirty years' experience and a life study in training the voice. They contain no superfluous exercises, and omit no essential ones.

This work is not intended to supersede the instruction of a master, but will materially aid both Teacher and Pupil in the cultivation and development of the voice, and supply a want long felt by those engaged in tuition.

The Exercises are written in all keys, with the most simple accompaniments, so that the student is not troubled to transpose them.

For further information, reference must be made to the author's concise and instructive Preface.

PRICE 1/6 NET.

London:

ROBERT COCKS & CO.,

6. NEW BURLINGTON STREET, W.,

Music Publishers to H.M. the Queen and H.R.H. the Prince of Wales.

Agents for the United States of America:

EDWARD SCHUBERTH & CO., New York.

— 25 —

Melodious Vocal Studies,

WITH

Easy Pianoforte Accompaniments.

BY

ANGELO MASCHERONI.

Price 2s. 6d. net.

LONDON:

ROBERT COCKS & CO.,

6, NEW BURLINGTON STREET, W.

Music Publishers to H.M. the Queen and H.R.H. the Prince of Wales.

AGENTS FOR THE UNITED STATES OF AMERICA:

EDWARD SCHUBERTH & CO., New York.

www.ingramcontent.com/pod-product-compliance
Lightning Source LLC
Chambersburg PA
CBHW022121090426
42743CB00008B/954
* 9 7 8 1 4 7 3 3 3 0 4 2 9 *

My Burning City

poems by

Arthur Kayzakian

Finishing Line Press
Georgetown, Kentucky

My Burning City

ISBN 979-8-88838-253-0 First Edition

ACKNOWLEDGMENTS

Gratitude for the editors of the journals who published some form of these poems:

The Southern Review: "The Craftsman"
Michigan Quarterly Review: "Synonyms for Maps"
Witness Magazine: "When We Fled Iran"
Prairie Schooner: "Rain," & "Armenian Folk Dance, 1915"
Southern Humanities Review: "Exiled to Los Angeles" (formerly "Exiled in Los Angeles")
Taos Journal of International Poetry & Art: "Anniversary"
Nat. Brut Magazine: "Translation" (Also published in We Were Not Alone: A Community Bulding Art-Works Anthology)
Anatolios Magazine: "Sonnet of My Grandfather the Original Lightning," "Exiled: Los Angeles" (formerly Exiled to Los Angeles)
Versions of this chapbook have been finalists for the Locked Horn Press Chapbook Prize, Two Sylvias Press Chapbook Prize, the C.D. Wright Prize, the Sunken Garden Poetry Prize, and the Black River Chapbook Competition, and won the PS Strousse Award for his poems published in the Spring 2020 issue of *Prairie Schooner.*

Publisher: Leah Huete de Maines
Editor: Christen Kincaid
Cover Art: Deborah Eater
Author Photo: Andy Smith
Cover Design: Elizabeth Maines McCleavy

Order online: www.finishinglinepress.com
also available on amazon.com

Author inquiries and mail orders:
Finishing Line Press
PO Box 1626
Georgetown, Kentucky 40324
USA

Table of Contents

Իմ Վառվող Քաղաքը

(My Burning City)

իմ վառվող քաղաքը

شهر سوخته من

(my burning city)

How we made it here I cannot say.

Sonnet of My Grandfather the Original կայծակ

My name in Armenian used to mean priest. At the gate
a guard raised his gun, *too many priests here*—forced
to contort his name before Tehran, my grandfather
changed it to electricity, bolted it across the border.
Now my name means lightning. The gloom around
the electrons of my name carry the charge of an empty
chair, the volt of a girl who sketches a sky dead
without birds. My grandfather held loss for his name.
It is a story of a man whose name became a ghost,
who tucked the bones of his last name in a duffle bag
and shuffled his feet to freedom. His body an asylum
for his missing name, which followed him like a phantom
longing for a tower of souls. All because he said lightning.
His head a trumpet blowing out an anthem of sparks.

Maps

After Brandon Melendez

fence | an imaginary line | a signature of victory at the expense of a skull | a translator of fields | a traitor of grass | the color green reminding me of my executed friends | paintings that lie | paintings that lie down | paintings that lie down in the rhythm of victory | victory victory victory | an invention to value document over blood | i call up a dead friend on a disconnected line | a partition between a dream and an obliterated collar bone | a mechanism for trade | zinc for laughter | fire for jokes | a geopolitical divide that supports a wall | the un-shingled rooftop festered with pigeons | the opposite of joy | antithesis to holding hands | to force queerness as a definition of distance | as in *man, you're gay* or *don't be so queer* | as in a line denying strangeness from beauty | a strange boundary | can i please have some water | a phantom rule that promotes mortgage | an urge to surge a needle in the vein | a distinction of history etched in dye | a king traced in dark laces of laughter | a president who clears a path through a sea of people | a contract stained with tea | a voided tree lot piled with wood | a city crawling over a land | my dead friends leave a message on a disconnected line | a sudden wave of a flag on a horse | the air cancelling the trespass of bullets

Please Ask

the pomegranate, split open

at the center of the dinner table
with red seeds glowing from its peel,

what happened to the Armenians?

Exiled: Los Angeles

We fled from green oil tanks and the scent of chemicals,
from fire bluster and windows rattled by gunfire.

We fled to make poems out of cemeteries
and write prose out of psalms.

Here, our windows are stained with promise.
Our prayers are made of glass.

From a confiscated garden infested with guards,
we fled to an army of daffodils.

We fled and we fled from Allah
burning in the trees, from gutted staircases

and swollen buildings sinking to the sand.
We fled from the parade of sirens.

Here, at night, dogs bark in the junkyard.
Our hands up against the wall,

We have been taught we die without one another.
What do we know of love?

Rain

After he hugs his family goodbye
        he passes umbrellas and park benches,

sees the edge of a vexed flower petal and thinks,
        the flower is a man off to war.

Without looking back,
        he can hear his children kicking

laughter in and out of him.
        His wife's throat, a gleam of sandlight.

Fifteen years later,
        rain beats out a puddle in the shape of his body.

Anniversary

Who, after all, speaks today of the annihilation of the Armenians?
—Adolf Hitler

In Armenia
one night a year for the dead
some wear black headscarves
lay flowers around the cenotaph
kneel before the sky and pray
to honor rainclouds
that never rained
that stacked on one another
rattled and dissipated
without notice.

Diaspora

On the corner of 110th
and Normandie,
a man plays the
harmonica, an empty
guitar case beside
him. *I'm Sokrat,*
and my next song is called
Home.
His breath
swelling the crowd
with his song. The people
clap, the man bows,
this song belonged to my ancestors
whose art I carry
in my blood.
Some nod,
some toss a handful
of coins
into his guitar case
and move on.

The Toast

When my lover raises her glass,
her blood rushes to the age of seven—

when she hid under the kitchen table
from soldiers in green uniforms who broke down her door,

and dragged her brother out of the house.
In June, they returned to her doorway, the guard,

with one arm behind his back,
knelt before her and said *I have a gift for you.*

Then held a skull in front of her
and blew over the right eye socket,

out droned a low hum
like the inside of a seashell

the guard looked up with a smirk,
I've made a flute for you.

We Waited

beneath the ravine
an old shack stacked with chainsaws and wood

the darkness smelled of chalk crawling with pine
our teeth chattered from the cold

and behold the hours to come
the galloping horses laced with burgundy riders

thumping overhead and though ceiling dust
sprinkled on our faces we waited in the floor boards

hoarded with old wood
the whisper of guards negotiating our capture

we listened to their voices under hot cocoa
pressed to their lips they sipped and sipped

with small talk sweet we could see
through the cracks men with graycoats

jacked with guns *thank you for the pleasantries*
and let us know if you see one coming your way

we hid from their voices that sparked in the dark
like electric omens of light

we stood close to our silence
under the floor with centipedes and roaches

scattered across our faces tingled our lips
as they passed

տուն (home)

The night I kissed my father on his cheek,

his smile,

from a charcoal Armenian, hard Armenian
glazed with the scent of smoke and bravado,

softened.

Not even silence has a name for that.

Geometry

The shape depends on the height of the human—
being my grandfather was not a tall man,

the top of the box took the form of his shoulders,
which carried my mother as a child.

It was unlike my grandfather to lie
in a hard-wooden coffin but he did.

The curves of thick timber from lid
to base ran angle-to-angle;

the mortician called the box a "polygon"—
a hexagon with six sides.

He said the head space was narrow
and the contours of the case were padded

with velvet: it reminded me of the color
our home turned during the day

when the sun slipped through the window,
how difficult it was to crawl through the corridors

before he lifted me in his arms.
How could this coffin hold such a man?

The Craftsman

my father carved wood
he laid the tree bark on a flat table
gretchcut the chainsaw through the grain
he made caskets and rifles
for men who unbuttoned their graycoats
sat on barstools ordering drink after drink
the surface of the lake rippled
from bombs dropped on the dark edges of town
one day the men in graycoats
knocked on my father's door
and asked him to kneel before the empire
I write this for you father
in the shed of your workshop
beside a pile of wood

Faith

You bite your nails,
search for a prayer in your fingers,

live in a two-story house with a green lawn,
but homeland is your mother's voice.

Some days the mind is a silver braid of water,
other days it jangles like a box of knives.

So you search your dresser,
look for your pills

scratch a nickel on a lottery ticket
for ecstasy, for a scrape of God.

Vespers

I pray I pray I pray till my sweat tastes of limefire;
till I measure what I've done
by the groundswell of flies that pepper my meat.
How we fall on a small earth.
My heart: a fence full of padlocks.
A needle of God in my arm last night,
even when it eats my brain,
even when it eats my creed,
I pray till my blood tastes of limefire, I pray I pray.
Bread Crumbs. Pigeons
resting on the red tongue of my nightdress.
In the green night, I see you, grandfather,
for this is how the dead blacken a piano.
It rains, as if heaven crashes, it rains.
And in the cigarette, I savor my burning city.

my [ ] is

asylum

history and its redcoat of time
my oath to the road
a wall scar from a taken painting
a box of police reports
a drumbeat fighting the hang of time
a window of falling bombs
a chart of redacted names
a tower of laughter
red pressed into trees
daughter to my water slang
thin run of a sunlit child
the syrup of flag blood
torpid velocity of a dark stain
the dance of bandana and fire
resisting arrest by a chain of flowers
a reflection of trees lost in a mirror
the stranger who stole my skeleton
a subversion of radio farsi
a quorum of birds

Reading with My Father

My father used to say a book is the song
of the body,

the way he scraped the sound out
of each word before he turned the page.

That a book smells
like plywood beneath the hot sun of Abadan.

He sat at the edge of my bed,
held the spine

and read as if the inside of a rock is made of dreams.

My father, who after reading to me each night,
loved to shut his door, turn off the lights

and sing to himself.

When We Fled Iran

this morning i pray
for the back of my father's hand
a map to manhood
across my face

when the air was raided with chemical
we sang from the jugular

i stood up to my father's hand
i watched his hand fall back
the shame i feel for standing up
for my failure to locate my country
in my father

Instructions for Survival

1. Wait until the phone rings in the middle of the night.

2. Disconnect it and say hello as if you are looking through a window.

3. Remove the painting from the wall and listen to the imprint it leaves behind.

4. Research the word silence.

5. Experiment the sound of invasion by knocking on the door.

6. Tell yourself mirrors are not subversive.

7. Read a map like a poem and see if it won't catch on fire.

8. Research the word erasure.

9. Look at the stain on the wall left from the painting you removed.

10. When the phone rings open the door in your hello before you answer.

Nocturnal

a strange thing when **i** changed the dial on the radio noise qu**a**ntu**m**
intercepted channel light bending through the window mirror
the atla**s** **o**f a skull mirror ga**t**her**i**ng shrapnel off the soon to be
bu**r**i**ed** sang the voice coiled in the speaker the same metallic that
scratched the back **of** runaways gutting underneath **b**arbed f**e**nces
as all my senses runn**ing** through my hands a jolt of freedom when
i help a cricket out the sink j**u**st the**n** a little friend **s**catt**e**rs across
th**e** wall i**n** its acceptance of crawling lost this is a pretext this signal
a legion of sirens is how I bargain with grief

Armenian Folk Dance, 1915

A man and woman hide in their home
to dance amid lit candles.

He kneels as she twirls
around him.

She raises both arms in the half-
light, and the shadow of her hands—

a bird in flight—brushes the wall.

If this were any other day, she would
clap to the beat of the drum.

She tip toes to keep quiet
from the crows outside the window

roosting upon crucifixes
that go on, row after row.

Tehran

Do you recall Iran? Outside our apartment
the b*rracka-brracka* cracked the air open.

The sound split the wind in half when it echoed
down the street, and leaves tumbled to the ground.

You shut windows and closed the blinds.
Do you remember footsteps near the door?

Turning the lights off you crouched next to me,
it's okay, it's okay, the parade is coming, coming to town.

The drums rolled from the edge of the city,
and the earth glowed through the blinds.

But that day you knelt and held my hands
through sand, through dust, through glass,

through drums that passed our street.
Together we climbed here. Up the parade

of bodies to outlive. Now our laughter happens, though
we know where hell came from: it fell from the sky.

Dear Invader

•

Last night I heard your horn warbling in my head.
I slept like a deep river in a Russian eye.
You scorched a war name on my skull
in Armenian, we call these nightmares *Chakata Gir.*

•

I know you've lost everything you love, and perhaps
you perceive me as a threat—

when you buried us down, we danced through a hole in the sun
in our reach for America.

We crossed the untenable sea like an arrowhead of birds.

•

Tell me Invader,
how does it feel to know you swallowed your faith?
Your stomach acid eating at your prayers.
And so, we both know—the night you burst through my door,

the night you want so desperately to redden me
with the absence in your gut—you've lost everything you love.

•

I know your desire: to pulverize us into a calligraphy of artifacts.
So you draw maps on the carcass of our bodies—propped up
behind a glass wall you call school:

"Here are the Armenians. They were quarantined like a silo of sick birds
when they couldn't weather the destiny of change."

•

All because we know you've lost everything
you love.

That hole inside you, the size of a bomb
you carry around like a heavy
bag of ghosts.

•

No matter how many houses you vaporize,
how many houses you raid,

we sing from the jugular.

We sing until you feel our terror
sting

through the walls of the homes you took.

•

So come and get us

because you—like us—wake in the morning,
walk to the sink and look in the mirror

while trying not to fall through the empty lake inside you.

Translation

as in the night that wrecked my hands, a city of crows daggered through the sky. as in a skull of complex nightmares, the black owl of my mouth, a box of dreams for strangling. as in hope, as in my mother's voice, as in we avoided the mouth of a door forced open. as in the quiet voice of god crashing through the lifeless, a separation: animal from spirit. from *kentanee* to *hokee*. as in salt turns an ocean nocturnal with its smallness. the night between us has a restless gap. as in birds flutter. as in cage, as in a wild hive of prayers under my breath. as in we live just one more breath with segments of light. as in we live in a city dragged to the sea by the hands of its night. as in the sugar of a dying language, the scent of ash and a bashed in door. as in smoke-rings blown from the mouth of a glorified general. as in river then a slice of jail. of wine stain, the torture of praying. as in history. as in we wait with white men for metal doors to slide open. as in instead of anger, we have flower petal weight on our shoulders. as in psychedelic. it's okay we smile. it's not okay we know: as in more red than music, more curtains dropped on our homes than nightfall. as in memory. as in the threaded rasp of my mother's voice cloaks the siren, she walks closer to me ever slowly dropping parts of her dark sky. as in instead of radio, a ghost picks up a stream, a frequency foreign to the ear. as in we are foreign stones who have turned to wishes without promise. as in we flee. we dance, moonwalk in our shadows. as in we fall. as in we fall through our mother's lies for safety. as in we live beneath the yellow death of sun, our language: a summer bomb mixed with extinction. as in i was delivered from war when my mother fired up the lie barricaded in her breast to save me. as in bandana. as in these days I feel ill-gotten, which is to say i'm rugged, as in I stare hard at a painting before I take it with me, as in my friends call me the armenian-persianist, as in an immigrant with a junkyard smile. as in my friends dress like wolves. as in joy has been swept to an aftermath of bodies, mangled. as in ill. as in cough from the small of my delicate sun. as in touch. as in we locked lips under the flicker of lights in a dim-walled hallway. as in my crime is not so much in denying my hunger, but the great extent i went to hide my ability for loss. as in ship. as in disembark. as in the english language. as in technology wheeling its way into my mouth until my broken native tongue spits out words in boats of abandon. as in the war. as in on us. as in the nights a city howls in honor of its body count. as in the cemetery has grown jealous of the city, and the evening tucked in its blade so the sunset could live.

Grass Stain

When my uncle knelt
at the tombstone,

the grass bowed before him,

and I remember the green
smudge on the right knee of his slacks.

He was the only man wearing white
at his father's funeral.

Sometimes I laugh when I think about it,

but then I recall the darkness
of that stain—

he must have put all his weight
to the ground when he knelt.

Dedications

This book would not be possible without my mother, who never stopped believing in me, my father, who is my source code for these poems, my brother, who helped me pull myself together, my uncle, who has been an inspiration for some of my work, my aunt who always told my mother I would not fall into darkness, my grandfather whose light fills my pen with strength each time I write, and my grandmother who gave up everything for me to reach my potential and write this book.

To my Higher Power who never led me astray, who saved my life, I owe everything to you, God.

To the healers: Chuck, Xavier, Danny (RIP), Bill, who asked me why I am angry with myself, and showed me a path to healing, thank you for helping me believe in myself. Theron, Tyler, Stephanie, Amanda, Jon, Nicole, and the Burbank Group with our late-night cigarette breaks at the table. Bradford Bancroft, who showed me how to access my light. Carolyn Wheeler for guiding me through my trauma.

To all my English and History teachers who helped me excavate my love for literature and writing: Mr. B from Burbank High Circa 1996, Mrs. McGrade from Wilson Circa 1992, Mr. MacFarlane from Wilson Circa 1992, Stephen Taylor from Glendale Community College Circa 2000, thank you for your guidance.

The Kanian Family. My Godfather Martik Kanian, Taleen Kanian, Artin Kanian. Carole Kanian, my Godmother, Rest in Power. Thank you for being my family.

To Leilani Hall, for guiding me during my time at CSUN, for introducing me to Terrance Hayes when you eloquently read "Lighthead's Guide to the Galaxy" on the first day of class, for the years of mentorship and guidance. Thank you, Dorothy Barresi, for showing me how all things are related to poetry. And to the CSUN faculty, including Mona Houghton, Rick Mitchell, Kate Haake, Jack Solomon, and Ranita

Chatterjee, thank you for the workshops, lectures, and discussions when I was your student—your expertise and generosity continue to inspire me.

To my CSUN Creative Writing cohort who inspired me during our time together, thank you for the wonderful memories. Sanam Shamiri, Alyssa Skalissa, Neda Levi, Sean Pessin, Trista Rista, Eric Barnhart, Robin Jewel Smith, Cyrus Sepahbodi, David Gale, Jamie Bezerra, Kim Young, Phil Chang, Davic Morck, Susana Aguilar-Mercano, Dylan Altman, Katie, McMahon, Alejandra Lucero Canaan, Kate Martin George Fekaris, and all my fellow CSUN classmates.

To my SDSU MFA family, these poems would not exist without you. Ilya Kaminsky for the inspirational years in San Diego, for showing me how to bite into my nouns. Sandra Alcosser on how to follow the image, for conversations about life as a poet. This book is a result of your faith in me. Katie Farris, I was your student who never got a chance to take your class. Thank you for our conversations and friendship, your creativity inspires me. Sherwin Bitsui, for asking me about my homeland, which I am still trying to write my way through. Blas Falconer, for spending countless hours working with me on poems. Steven Paul Mitchell, for the brilliant conversations about magic realism. Meagan Marshall for your light, energy, brilliance, and of course, the Living Writers Series. William Nericcio, Circular of Ruins, and Phillip Serrato, Chicanx Literature. Mary Garcia, for your guidance. Ashley Vorraro, for the many conversations between classes.

To my SDSU MFA cohort, you have helped me shape my voice with the many conversations, readings, and workshops during and post MFA, for which I am fortunate. Hari Alluri, Karla Cordero, Kevin Dublin, Garrett Bryant, Janel Spencer, Jennifer Ruby, Alyssabeth K-Bzka, Erica Blunt, Theo Niekras, Ana Bosch, and to all my fellow classmates, thank you for your warm friendship, amazing feedback, collaboration on projects, late night hookah hangouts, and our continued work together.

To the many poets and professionals that I continue to learn from, I am in awe of your talent and wisdom. Zephyr Poets crew, Alene Terzian-Zeitounian, Arminé Iknadossian, Mary Angelino, and Shahe Mankerian, for all your rigorous and honest feedback on poems, for your friendship and love. Lory Bedikian, for the music in my manuscript, for guiding me toward my soul when revising my book, for the thousand conversations about life and craft, for your warm friendship and undeniable generosity. Armen Davoudian, for your friendship and conversations about poems. Sophia Armen, for recognizing my work in your publication, for the few but real conversations. Piotr Florczyk, for our many conversations and our time at AWP. Chris Abani and the Las Brujas workshop in 2017, for asking me, "when was the first time you lost your innocence?" for writing from the wound. Cynthia Dewi Oka, for our many conversations about poetry over bomb ass food. Nicole Sealey for bringing awareness to the parameters in making a cento. Cyrus Sepahbodi, thank you for believing in me, for the countless conversations about poetry, for the typewriter session under the Magnolia tree, for the five solid years of Lamp Light Poetry with David Gale, and for helping me build the courage to embrace my ghost. To Ruth Christopher Sepahbodi, thank you for your talent and our many conversations about poetry that continue to inspire me. To my Mad Mouth crew, David Gale, Maya Alexandria, Dameika Thomas, working on poetry with you has been the light I needed during the pandemic. Meri Tumanyan, for the many years of friendship, my workshop roll dawg. Beth Marquez, for your friendship, inspiration, talent, and our amazing conversations about poetry. To Amy Schroeder for your generosity in reading an earlier version of this manuscript. Arlin Vartanian, my dear friend and poet, who suggested I write in free verse twenty years ago, I cannot thank you enough. Shant Shahoian, Tanya Baronian, our laughter, anger, our humor. SDSU, CSUN, GCC, PCC, COC, and Chaffey College for your support and warmth. Janet Frnzyan, for your deep friendship and support, I am forever grateful to have you in my life. Ara Arzumanian, for the many days we spent writing poems at GCC. William Archilla, Raychelle Heath, Carrie Mar, Miguel Ángeles, Tara Sarath, Faria Ali,

Hari Alluri, Aurora Masum-Javed, Elizabeth Hassler, Laura Jew, thank you for your warmth and friendship in building community for our many workshops.

To these poets, I owe my deepest gratitude in helping me shape my manuscript into My Burning City. Blas Falconer, for spending countless hours helping me polish these poems. Kaveh Akbar, for your friendship, for showing me how to introduce silence into my work. Brendan Constantine, for the many workshops and how you've inspired me, for inviting me to your home and spending time with me sorting out poems. Layli Long Soldier, Diana Khoi Nguyen, Daisy Fried, Cynthia Dewi Oka, Rosebud Ben-Oni, Joseph Rios, Sara Borjas (for the inspiring conversations), Karla Cordero, Hari Alluri for your brilliant and generous workshop intensives. Seema Reza and the Community Building Artworks (CBAW) team, where many of the poems in this book were born, thank you for the weekly workshops that saved my life during the pandemic and helped me expand my writing in ways that I am still learning from and holding within.

The International Armenian Literary Alliance (IALA) board of directors, advisory board members and friends who are also brilliant artists and professionals—Lola Koundakjian, J.P. Der Boghossian, Shahé Mankerian, Nancy Agabian, Levon Golendukhin, you have given me a home to speak from, a platform to raise my voice. Olivia Katrandjian, for founding IALA, our home, for pointing out that Vartan Mamikonian needs a book of his own—this changed the course of my manuscript. Gregory Djanikian, for your friendship and mentorship and our conversations. Mashinka Firunts Hakopian, Lory Bedikian, Alan Semerdjian, Peter Balakian, Tatevik Ayvazyan, Aida Zilelian, and the whole community we've grown, thank you for the communities you help build.

To all my childhood friends and ones I've crossed paths with for a brief moment in time, who have in some way inspired and supported me to become the person I am today: Artin Vartanian, Ed Cholakian, Artin Cholakian, Emily Jenny Cholakian, Chantel Cholakian, Artin

Nazarian, Armen Zadoorian, Alen Kazaryan, Mike Akopyan, David Markosyan, Fred Avanossian, Dvin Bahariance, Edita Baburova, Sandy Kochova, Eddie Andonian, Annie Hartounian, Erika Hartounian, Teni Hartounian, Andrew Hartounian, Arne Hartounian, Nairi Ayvazyan, Leona Balalian, Hiuro, Zareh Karimian aka Reno, Teni Karimian, Sassoun Davoodian, Shaunt Kodaverdian, Sabina Ohanessian, Raffi Barsamian, Karen Davoodian, Adam Davoodian, Dro aka Triple D, Dro Telmi, Irma Telmi, Andy Kushner, Narbeh Der Gevorkian, Irene HayDer Gevorkian Armen Asefi, Val Asefi, Pedro Madadian aka P-Dawg, AC, Cap Z, R-Mean, David aka Voicebox, Human, Bei Ru, Sassoun Ashoughian, Joseph Dunlap, Chris Choi, Kixxo Rios, Greg Alexanian, Annie Hamamchian, Prince Troy, aka Little, aka Cousin, Sam Babayan, James Cho, Andy Smith, Valerie Adissi, Naham. Rest in Power Ara Lux & Eddie Movsesian. Thank you for the times we spent together—our experiences have shaped me in ways

Editor-in-Chief Mai Der Vang, Judge Carmen Jimenez Smith, and Anhinga Press at Fresno State University for the labor of deep reading my work, for the vote of confidence in selecting The Book of Redacted Paintings as a finalist for the Philip Levine Prize.

My deepest gratitude to Black Lawrence Press Editor-in Chief, Diane Goettel for working closely with me to ensure this book makes it to the shelves. To the Immigrant Writing Series editors, Abayomi Animashaun, Sun Yung Shin, Rigoberto Gonzalez, and Ewa Chrusciel, thank you for honoring my work by selecting it for the inaugural Immigrant Writing Series—this means the world to me.

Anita Walinska, my deepest gratitude goes to you and the Gorky Foundation. Thank you for your kind note. I hope your letter reaches the hands of whoever has "The Portrait of Anna Walinska" in their possession.

To those redacted from being named, I know there are many who I fail to recognize in these notes who have in some way shaped me as an artist, I hope this warm thank you reaches through the shadows to you.

End Notes

What follows is a record of excerpts and images from the poets and artists who have influenced my work. In some poems, I was inspired by a line while in others it may be form.

Sonnet of My Grandfather the Original կայծակ

The line "It is a story of a man whose name became a ghost," is influenced by Terrance Hayes' "it is the story of a son / whose father is a ghost" from *American Sonnets For My Past And Future Assassins.*

my [   ] is

The line "the syrup of flag blood" is an imitation and response to Terrance Hayes' "The mix of flag blood & surprise blurring the eyes, a flare" from *American Sonnets For My Past And Future Assassins.*

Synonyms for Maps

The form for this poem is inspired by the poet Brandon Melendez's poem "Synonyms for Border."

When We Fled Iran

The line "this morning i pray" is borrowed from Joy Harjo's title, "This Morning I Pray for My Enemies" in *Conflict Resolution for Holy Beings.*

Arthur Kayzakian is the winner of the 2021 inaugural Black Lawrence Immigrant Writing Series for his collection, *The Book of Redacted Paintings*, which was also selected as a finalist for the 2021 Philip Levine Prize for Poetry. He is the recipient of the 2023 creative writing fellowship from the National Endowment for the Arts. He also won the PS Straosse award for poems in *Prairie Schooner* and the Finishing Line Press Open Chapbook Competition for, *My Burning City.* He serves as the Poetry Chair for the International Armenian Literary Alliance (IALA). His work has appeared in several publications, including *The Adroit Journal, Portland Review, Chicago Review, Cincinnati Review, The Southern Review, Michigan Quarterly Review,* and *Witness Magazine.*

www.ingramcontent.com/pod-product-compliance
Lightning Source LLC
Chambersburg PA
CBHW022124090426
42743CB00008B/997